THE OPIOID EPIDEMIC OF AMERICA

:The uses of Naloxone,side effects and why parents should administer it for their children

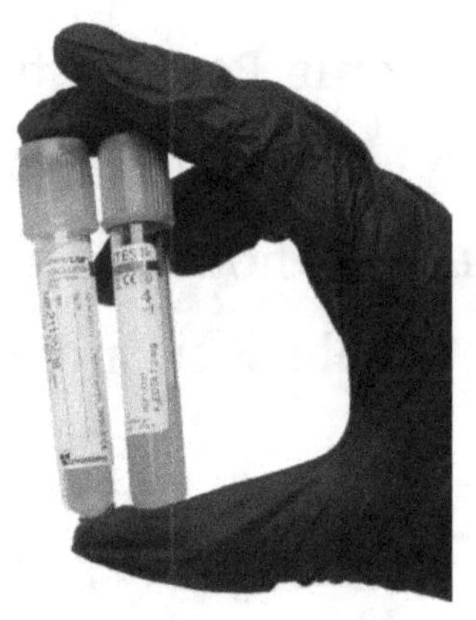

Dr. Sam A. Malvin

TABLE OF CONTENT

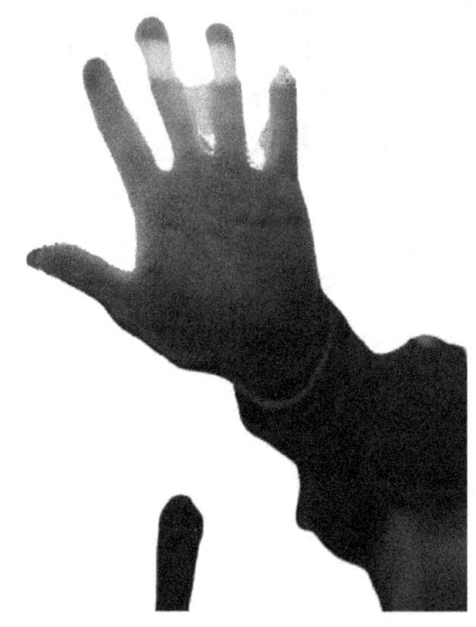

Introduction

The Biden administration has called on schools in the United States to stock naloxone, an opioid overdose reversal drug, in an effort to combat the rising number of overdose deaths among teens.

In a joint letter to educators, Dr. Rahul Gupta, the Director of the White House Office of National Drug Control Policy, and Miguel Cardona, the US Secretary of Education, emphasized the importance of having naloxone readily available in schools to prevent and respond to opioid overdoses.

Naloxone, often sold under the brand name Narcan, is a medication that can reverse the effects of an opioid overdose by blocking the opioids' effects on the brain and restoring normal breathing. It is most effective when administered as soon as signs of an overdose appear. Importantly, naloxone only works on individuals who have opioids in their system and does not have adverse effects when given to someone who hasn't taken opioids.

The US Food and Drug Administration (FDA) recently approved over-the-counter use of Narcan, making it more accessible. The manufacturer of the OTC Narcan, Emergent BioSolutions, has lowered the medication's price for community groups, first responders, state and local governments, and harm reduction groups to $41 per two-dose carton.

The initiative to make naloxone available in schools is a response to the alarming increase in overdose deaths among teens, with more than 5,000 children and teens dying from overdoses involving fentanyl in the past two decades.

In 2021, there were over 1,550 pediatric deaths from fentanyl, more than 30 times the number in 2013 when the surge of overdose deaths involving synthetic opioids began in the US.

The majority of pediatric deaths from fentanyl have been among teenagers aged 15 to 19. The push to stock naloxone in schools is part of a broader effort by the White House to address the dangers of illicit drugs like fentanyl, reduce the stigma around mental health, and strengthen community safety.

The Biden administration's Youth Substance Use Prevention Summit aims to raise awareness of these issues. The US Centers for Disease Control and Prevention (CDC) supports the effort to bring naloxone to schools and is committed to working with communities to prevent youth substance use and reduce overdoses.

Schools are seen as integral to the success of local Drug-Free Communities, and the Department of Education is dedicated to helping schools establish positive school cultures, implement evidence-based drug prevention strategies, and provide staff with the tools and training to respond to drug-induced health emergencies.

The opioid crisis is an urgent and deeply concerning issue that affects communities across the United States. In this book, we will delve into this crisis, aiming to shed light on the situation and the actions we can take to address it.

Additionally, we'll explore naloxone, a life-saving tool that holds immense importance in these trying times.

Chapter 1

Understanding the Opioid Crisis

The Opioid Epidemic in the United States

The opioid epidemic in the United States is a public health crisis that has claimed millions of lives. Opioids are a variety of drugs that include prescription painkillers, heroin, and fentanyl. They are used to treat pain, but they can also be addictive and lead to overdose and death.

The opioid epidemic began in the late 1990s with the overprescribing of prescription painkillers.

Over the next decade, opioid overdose deaths increased steadily. In 2017, more than 47,000 people in the United States died from opioid overdoses, making it the leading cause of accidental death among Americans under the age of 50.

The Rising Threat to Teenagers

Teenagers are particularly vulnerable to the opioid epidemic. They are more likely to experiment with drugs and take risks. They are also more likely to be exposed to opioids through friends, family members, or social media.

The rate of opioid overdose deaths among teenagers has increased significantly in recent years.

In 2017, more than 1,500 teenagers died from opioid overdoses, a 56% increase from 2015.

The Role of Naloxone in Overdose Prevention

What is Naloxone?

Naloxone has a brand name called Narcan, is a drug used to reverse an opioid overdose. It functions by blocking the effects of opioids on the brain.

Naloxone is available in a variety of forms, including nasal sprays, auto-injectors, and injectable solutions. Naloxone is generally administered by anyone, regardless of medical training.

How Naloxone Works

When a person takes an opioid, the drug binds to opioid receptors in the brain. This blocks pain signals and produces feelings of euphoria. However, opioids can also slow down breathing and heart rate, which can lead to overdose and death.

Naloxone works by displacing opioids from opioid receptors. This restores normal breathing and heart rate and reverses the overdose.

The Importance of Timely Intervention
The sooner naloxone is administered, the more effective it is at reversing an overdose.

If you suspect someone is experiencing an opioid overdose, call 911 immediately. While you wait for help to arrive, you can administer naloxone if available.

To administer naloxone nasal spray, follow these steps:

1. The cap should be removed from the nasal spray.

2. Insert the tip of the nozzle into one nostril.

3. Release the dose by pressing the plunger firmly

4. Repeat steps 2 and 3 in the other nostril.

To administer naloxone auto-injector, follow these steps:

1. Remove the cap from the auto-injector.

2. Place the auto-injector firmly against the person's outer thigh, just above the knee.

3. Press the plunger firmly.

4. Hold the auto-injector in place for 5 seconds.

Chapter 2

Recognizing the Opioid Crisis

Origins and Causes

The opioid crisis in the United States has its roots in the late 1990s, when pharmaceutical companies began aggressively marketing prescription painkillers as safe and effective for treating chronic pain. Doctors began prescribing these drugs at alarming rates, even for mild pain conditions.

Over time, many people became addicted to prescription painkillers.

As they developed tolerance to the drugs, they needed to take higher and higher doses to achieve the same effects. This led to a shift towards heroin use, which is a cheaper and more potent opioid.

The opioid crisis has been fueled by a number of factors, including: Aggressive marketing of prescription painkillers by pharmaceutical companies.

- Overprescribing of prescription painkillers by doctors.
- Lack of access to evidence-based treatment for pain and addiction.
- The stigma associated with addiction.

- Social and economic factors, such as poverty and unemployment.

The Impact on Families

The opioid crisis has had a devastating impact on families across the United States. Several families have lost their loved ones to this crisis, and they have struggled to cope with the emotional and financial burdens of addiction.

Children who grow up in households with opioid addiction are at increased risk for a number of negative outcomes, including:

- Physical and emotional abuse
- Neglect
- Developmental delays
- Mental health problems
- Substance abuse

The Alarming Rise of Overdose Deaths Among Teens

Opioid overdose deaths among teenagers have increased dramatically in recent years. In 2017, more than 1,500 teenagers died from opioid overdoses, a 56% increase from 2015.

Statistics and Trends

The following statistics illustrate the alarming rise of opioid overdose deaths among teenagers:

In 2017, the rate of opioid overdose deaths among teenagers was 3.2 per 100,000, up from 2.1 per 100,000 in 2015.

The increase in opioid overdose deaths among teenagers has been driven primarily by fentanyl, a synthetic opioid that is 50 to 100 times more potent than morphine.

Fentanyl is often mixed with other drugs, such as heroin and cocaine, without the user's knowledge. This can lead to accidental overdoses.

Social and Economic Factors

A number of social and economic factors have contributed to the rise of opioid overdose deaths among teenagers, including:

- Poverty
- Unemployment
- Lack of access to healthcare
- Exposure to violence

- Trauma

Teenagers who live in poverty are more likely to use opioids than teenagers who come from wealthier backgrounds. They are also more likely to have difficulty accessing treatment for addiction.

Unemployment and lack of access to healthcare can also lead to opioid use among teenagers. Teenagers who are unemployed are more likely to feel hopeless and stressed, which can make them more vulnerable to addiction. Teenagers who lack access to healthcare may have difficulty getting the treatment they need for pain, which can lead them to turn to opioids.

Violence and trauma can also increase the risk of opioid use among teenagers. Teenagers who are exposed to violence, either as victims or witnesses, are more likely to experience mental health problems, such as depression and anxiety. These mental health problems can increase the risk of opioid use and addiction.

Chapter 3

Naloxone - The Life-Saving Medication

Understanding Naloxone: The Drug that Reverses Overdoses

Let's delve into the world of Naloxone, also known as Narcan, a medicine designed to reverse the effects of opioid overdoses. Naloxone's magic lies in its ability to block the dangerous impact of opioids on the brain.

Naloxone comes in different forms, such as nasal sprays, auto-injectors, and injectable solutions.

The good news is that anyone, regardless of medical training, can use it.

Varieties and How to Administer

Naloxone comes in three main forms:

1. Nasal Spray: The most common version is the nasal spray. It's user-friendly and can be administered by just about anyone. To use it, remove the cap, insert the nozzle into a nostril, and press the plunger to deliver the dose. Do the same to the other nostril.

2. Auto-Injector: The auto-injector is a nifty device that automatically injects Naloxone into the thigh.

To use it, remove the cap, place it on the person's outer thigh (just above the knee), press the plunger firmly, and hold the device in place for 5 seconds.

3. Injectable Solution: Typically, healthcare pros use injectable Naloxone in hospitals or clinics, but it's also available as a pre-filled syringe for emergencies. In this case, you inject the medication into the thigh or buttock muscle.

The Mechanism of Action

Naloxone acts by pushing opioids away from their spots on opioid receptors in the brain. This helps to restore normal breathing and heart rate, effectively reversing the overdose.

How Naloxone Reverses Opioid Overdoses

Opioids latch onto opioid receptors in the brain, which relieves pain and produces a euphoric sensation. But the dark side is that opioids can slow down breathing and heart rate, potentially leading to overdose and even death. Naloxone's superhero act is to boot opioids off these receptors, returning breathing and heart rate to normal, thus saving the day.

Safety and Effectiveness

Naloxone is a champ when it comes to safety and effectiveness. It doesn't come with any serious side effects, and it can be used by people of all ages, including pregnant women and those with other medical conditions.

Studies have shown that Naloxone can reverse an opioid overdose in more than 90% of cases. It's a life-saver that's both safe and dependable.

Chapter 4: Uses of naloxone

Why Naloxone is so essential

Naloxone is incredibly crucial because it has the power to save lives when someone is going through an opioid overdose. These overdoses can happen unexpectedly and anywhere. Naloxone is a safe and effective medicine that can turn an overdose around, preventing a tragic outcome.

Potential Overdose Scenarios

There are various situations where someone might experience an opioid overdose. Here are a few common scenarios:

1. Alone with Opioids: Sometimes, people use opioids by themselves, and if things go wrong, Naloxone can come to the rescue.

2. Mixing with Other Substances: Some folks mix opioids with other substances like alcohol or benzodiazepines. This combination can be very dangerous, and Naloxone can help reverse the overdose.

3. Accidental Overdose: People who take prescription opioids may accidentally take too much due to a misunderstanding or miscalculation. Naloxone can be a lifesaver in such cases.

4. Illicit Opioids: When someone uses illegal opioids like heroin or fentanyl, the risk of overdose is high, making Naloxone a critical tool in saving lives.

Naloxone in Different Places and settings

Naloxone isn't just for hospitals and doctors; it's useful in various settings to prevent opioid overdoses.
Here are some of those places:

Schools

Some schools now keep Naloxone on hand to address opioid overdoses among students. Overdoses can occur due to prescription opioid misuse, illegal drug use, or accidental exposure. Naloxone can make a real difference in schools.

Homes

If someone uses opioids at home, it's a good idea to have Naloxone readily available, for any emergency.

You can get Naloxone from a pharmacy or a local health organization.

Community Events

Events like concerts and festivals can be hotspots for opioid overdoses. Naloxone can be a lifesaver in such settings, preventing overdose-related deaths.

Public Places

Public areas like parks and restrooms can also be locations where opioid use occurs. Naloxone can be used here to prevent overdose deaths.

And beyond these places, Naloxone is used in hospitals, clinics, by law enforcement agencies, fire departments, homeless shelters, and drug treatment programs.

It's also becoming more accessible to the general public through community programs and pharmacies.

This is vital because opioid overdoses can happen anywhere, and having Naloxone available can truly save lives.

Chapter 4: Naloxone Administration

Recognizing the Signs of an Opioid Overdose

Below are some signs and symptoms of an opioid overdose:
- Loss of consciousness
- Slow or shallow breathing
- Blue lips or fingernails
- Cold and clammy skin
- Pinpoint pupils
- Vomiting
- Gurgling noises
- Seizures

If you see someone experiencing any of these signs or symptoms, call 911 immediately and administer naloxone if you have it.

Dosage and Methods of Administration

Naloxone is available in a variety of forms, including nasal spray, auto-injector, and injectable solution. The dosage of naloxone depends on the form of naloxone being used.

1. **Nasal spray**: The recommended dosage of naloxone nasal spray is 4 mg. If the person does not respond after 2-3 minutes, a second dose can be administered.

2. Auto-injector: The recommended dosage of naloxone auto-injector is 1 mg. If the person does not respond after 2-3 minutes, a second dose can be administered.

3. Injectable solution: The recommended dosage of naloxone injectable solution is 0.4 mg. If the person does not respond after 2-3 minutes, a second dose can be administered.

Tips for Effective Use

Here are some tips for effective use of naloxone:

- Administer naloxone as soon as possible after the overdose.

The sooner naloxone is administered, the more effective it is at reversing the overdose.

- If the person does not respond to the first dose of naloxone, administer a second dose after 2-3 minutes.
- Be with the person and monitor their breathing until help arrives.

Training and Education

It is important to learn how to use naloxone safely before using it. There are a number of training and education programs available. You can find naloxone training programs near you by searching online or by contacting your local public health department.

Resources and Training Programs

Here are some resources and training programs for naloxone:

- Harm Reduction Coalition: The Harm Reduction Coalition is a national organization that works to reduce the harms associated with drug use. They offer a variety of resources and training programs on naloxone.
- Naloxone Finder: Naloxone Finder is a website that helps people find naloxone near them.

- National Institute on Drug Abuse (NIDA): NIDA is a federal agency that supports research on drug use and addiction.

- They offer a variety of resources on naloxone, including training materials and a list of naloxone training providers.

- Centers for Disease Control and Prevention (CDC): The CDC is a federal agency that works to protect public health. They offer a variety of resources on naloxone, including training materials and a list of naloxone training providers.

Chapter 5: Potential Side Effects and Safety Considerations

Understanding Side Effects

Naloxone is a safe and effective medication, but it can cause some side effects. **The most common side effects of naloxone are:**

- Headache
- Dizziness
- Nausea
- Vomiting
- Sweating
- Goosebumps
- Muscle cramps
- Anxiety

These side effects are usually mild and go away on their own within a few minutes. However, if you experience any of these side effects, it is important to seek medical attention to rule out any other underlying medical conditions.

When to Seek Medical Assistance

If you experience any of the following side effects after administering naloxone, seek medical attention immediately:

- Difficulty breathing
- Chest pain
- Fast or irregular heartbeat
- Seizures
- Loss of consciousness

These side effects may be a sign of a serious medical condition, such as an overdose of another drug or a heart attack.

Legal and Ethical Considerations

Good Samaritan Laws

Good Samaritan laws protect people who help others in need from being sued. In the United States, all 50 states have a Good Samaritan law for naloxone. This means that you cannot be sued for administering naloxone to someone who is overdosing, even if they do not respond to the naloxone or if they experience side effects.

Stigma and Misconceptions

There is some stigma associated with naloxone use. Some people believe that naloxone is only used by people who use drugs, or that it enables people to use drugs more safely. However, these beliefs are false. Naloxone is a lifesaving medication that can be used by anyone to reverse an opioid overdose.

It is important to remember that opioid overdoses can happen to anyone, regardless of their age, race, ethnicity, or socioeconomic status. Naloxone is a tool that can save lives, and it should not be stigmatized.

Chapter 6: Preparing for the Unexpected

Naloxone Kits: What Should You Have on Hand

A naloxone kit should contain the following items:

- Naloxone nasal spray or auto-injector
- Instructions on how to use naloxone
- Gloves
- Barrier device for rescue breathing (e.g., pocket mask)

You can purchase naloxone kits from most pharmacies or online.

You can also obtain naloxone kits from some public health organizations and community programs.

Where to Obtain Naloxone Kits

Naloxone kits are available from the following sources:

- Pharmacies
- Public health organizations
- Community programs
- Online retailers

Talking to Children and Teens

It is important to talk to your children and teens about naloxone and opioid overdoses. These conversations should be age-appropriate and tailored to your child's level of understanding.

Below are some tips for talking to children and teens about naloxone:

- Start by explaining what opioid overdoses are and why they happen.
- Explain to them about naloxone and how it works.
- Let your child know that naloxone is a safe and effective way to reverse an opioid overdose.
- Answer any questions your child has about naloxone and opioid overdoses.
- Create an open and supportive environment where your child feels comfortable talking to you about drugs and addiction.

Age-Appropriate Discussions

The following are some age-appropriate discussions you can have with your children and teens about naloxone:

- Young children: For young children, you can focus on teaching them the signs and symptoms of an opioid overdose. You can also explain that there is a medicine called naloxone that can save someone's life if they are overdosing.
- Teenagers: For teenagers, you can provide more detailed information about naloxone and opioid overdoses. You can also discuss the risks of drug use and how to get help for addiction.

Creating an Open and Supportive Environment

It is important to create an open and supportive environment where your child feels comfortable talking to you about drugs and addiction.

Here are some tips:

- Listen to your child without judgment.
- Be honest and open with your child about your own experiences with drugs and addiction.
- Let your child know that you are there for them if they need help.

Chapter 7: Why Parents Should Administer Naloxone

Empowering Parents to Save Lives

Parents play a vital role in overdose prevention. They can talk to their children about the risks of drug use and addiction, and they can teach them about naloxone. Parents can also keep naloxone on hand in case their child or someone they know experiences an overdose.

A Parent's Role in Overdose Prevention

Parents can play a significant role in overdose prevention by:

- Talking to their children about the risks of drug use and addiction
- Teaching their children about naloxone
- Keeping naloxone on hand
- Monitoring their children for signs and symptoms of drug use
- Seeking help for their children if they need it

Fostering a Culture of Safety

Parents can also foster a culture of safety in their homes and communities by:

- Talking to their children about the importance of harm reduction
- Teaching the children how to make safe choices
- Supporting naloxone access and education programs
- Advocating for policies that promote overdose prevention

Personal Stories of Naloxone Success

There are many real-life accounts of naloxone use saving lives. Here is one example:

Sarah's Story

Sarah was a loving mother of two young children. She was also struggling with an opioid addiction. One day, Sarah overdosed on opioids at home. Her children were home at the time, and they called 911.

When the paramedics arrived, Sarah was unconscious and not breathing. They administered naloxone, and Sarah began to breathe again. Sarah was taken to the hospital, where she made a full recovery.

Sarah's story is a reminder that naloxone can save lives. It is also a reminder that parents should have naloxone on hand in case their child or someone they know experiences an overdose.

Chapter 8: Conclusion

The Urgent Need for Naloxone Awareness

The opioid crisis is a public health emergency that has claimed millions of lives. Naloxone is a safe and effective medication that can reverse an opioid overdose, but many people are not aware of it or do not have access to it.

It is important to raise awareness of naloxone so that people know how to use it to save lives. Naloxone should be widely available and affordable so that everyone has access to it in an emergency.

Joining the Effort to Combat the Opioid Crisis

There are many ways to join the effort to combat the opioid crisis and raise awareness of naloxone.

Here are a few ideas:

- Talk to your family and friends about naloxone and the opioid crisis.
- Donate to organizations that are working to prevent overdoses and provide naloxone access.
- Advocate for policies that promote overdose prevention and naloxone access.
- Get trained on how to administer naloxone.

- Keep naloxone on hand in case you or someone you know experiences an overdose.

Moving Forward

We need to work together to make naloxone more widely available and affordable. We also need to continue to raise awareness of naloxone and the opioid crisis. By working together, we can save lives and combat the opioid crisis.

Encouraging Naloxone Advocacy and Accessibility

There are a number of ways to encourage naloxone advocacy and accessibility.

Here are a few ideas:

- Contact your elected officials and urge them to support policies that promote naloxone access and overdose prevention.
- Support organizations that are working to make naloxone more widely available and affordable.
- Volunteer your time to help educate others about naloxone and the opioid crisis.
- Share information about naloxone on social media and other online platforms.

Hope for a Safer Future

By raising awareness of naloxone and making it more widely available, we can save lives and combat the opioid crisis. We can create a safer future for everyone.

Conclusion

The opioid crisis is a public health emergency, but there is hope. Naloxone is generally safe and effective medication that can reverse an opioid overdose. By working together to raise awareness of naloxone and make it more widely available, we can save lives and create a safer future for everyone.

questions and seek clarifications. Remember, communication is key in code reviews!

HOW TO CONDUCT EFFECTIVE CODE REVIEWS

Now that you know the components of a code review, let's discuss how to conduct effective code reviews. Here are a few tips to ensure your code reviews are practical learning sessions rather than nitpicking sessions:

- **Be specific**: Instead of saying, "This code is messy," provide specific examples and suggestions for improvement. For example, "Consider refactoring this function to improve readability by extracting repetitive logic into a separate helper function."

- **Focus on the big picture**: While it's important to catch small bugs, don't lose sight of the larger goals. Prioritize the

review based on the impact the changes
will have on the overall system.

- **Be respectful**: Remember, behind every
  line of code is a developer who poured their
  heart and soul into it. Be respectful and
  provide feedback in a professional and
  constructive manner.

- **Balance praise and critique**: It's easy to
  focus on the negatives, but don't forget to
  acknowledge and appreciate the positive
  aspects of the code. A well-placed
  compliment can go a long way in
  motivating and encouraging the developer.

- **Encourage dialogue**: Code reviews should
  be a collaborative process. Encourage the
  developer to ask questions, seek
  clarifications, and engage in meaningful
  discussions. This will foster a culture of
  learning and growth within the team.

By following these guidelines, you'll not only
improve the codebase but also create a positive
and supportive environment for your fellow
developers. Remember, code reviews are not just

about finding bugs; they're about building stronger teams and nurturing talent.

In the next chapter, we'll explore the role of a mentor in code reviews and how their guidance can elevate the entire process. So buckle up, grab your review checklist, and get ready to embark on a mentoring adventure!

Chapter 2 - Role of Mentor in Code Reviews

In this chapter, we will delve into the crucial role that mentors play in the code review process. Mentoring is not just about providing guidance and feedback; it is about fostering a positive and supportive environment that promotes learning and growth. A skilled mentor can turn a code review into a valuable mentoring opportunity for the mentee, helping them develop their skills and become better programmers.

THE IMPORTANCE OF MENTORING

Mentoring is a vital component of any successful code review process. It bridges the gap between theory and practice, providing mentees with real-world insights and practical advice. A mentor's role is not limited to pointing out mistakes or suggesting improvements; it is about helping the mentee understand the reasoning behind the feedback and guiding them towards finding their own solutions.

MENTORING RESPONSIBILITIES DURING A CODE REVIEW

1. **Setting Clear Expectations**: As a mentor, it is essential to establish clear expectations with the mentee before diving into the code review. Discuss the goals and objectives of the review, and ensure the mentee

understands what they should focus on and what is expected of them.

2. **Providing Constructive Feedback**: Feedback is the cornerstone of a successful code review. A mentor should provide feedback that is specific, actionable, and focused on improvement. Avoid vague or overly critical comments and instead offer suggestions and alternative approaches.

3. **Encouraging Self-Reflection**: A good mentor encourages the mentee to reflect on their own code and identify areas for improvement. Instead of spoon-feeding solutions, ask thought-provoking questions that prompt the mentee to think critically and find their own answers.

4. **Sharing Best Practices**: Mentors should share their knowledge and experience by highlighting best practices and industry standards. This could include recommending coding patterns, performance optimizations, or security considerations. By imparting this

knowledge, mentors help mentees level up their skills and become better programmers.

5. **Promoting Collaboration**: Code reviews shouldn't be a one-way street. Mentors should encourage collaboration and open communication between team members. Foster an environment where mentees feel comfortable asking questions, seeking clarification, and engaging in healthy discussions.

6. **Providing Emotional Support**: Learning from feedback can be challenging, especially for novice or mid-level programmers. A mentor should provide emotional support and reassurance during the code review process. Celebrate successes, acknowledge efforts, and guide mentees through any setbacks they may encounter.

MENTORSHIP AS A TWO-WAY STREET

While mentors have a crucial role to play in code reviews, it is equally important for mentees to actively participate and embrace the mentorship opportunity. Mentees should be open to feedback and willing to learn from more experienced team members. They should actively seek guidance, ask questions, and take ownership of their own development.

Remember, mentorship is a continuous process that extends beyond individual code reviews. Mentors should aim to build a lasting relationship with their mentees, providing ongoing support and guidance throughout their programming journey.

By embracing the role of mentor in code reviews, not only do we improve the quality of our code, but we also foster a culture of continuous learning and growth within our teams. So, let's grab our virtual mentoring capes and dive into the world of code reviews as mentoring opportunities!

Chapter 3 - Communication Skills

Communication is a vital skill in any professional setting, and code reviews are no exception. As a mentor, your role goes beyond just reviewing code - you are also responsible for guiding and assisting less experienced or newer programmers. This chapter will highlight the importance of effective communication during code reviews and provide tips on how to improve your communication skills as a mentor.

THE IMPORTANCE OF EFFECTIVE COMMUNICATION

When conducting a code review, it is crucial to communicate your feedback and suggestions clearly and effectively. Remember, the goal is not to criticize or belittle the programmer but to help them grow and improve their coding skills. Here are a few reasons why effective communication is essential during code reviews:

1. **Clarity**: Clear communication ensures that the mentee understands your feedback and suggestions accurately. Use simple and concise language, avoiding technical jargon that might confuse or overwhelm them.

2. **Openness**: Encourage an open and collaborative environment during code reviews. Be approachable and receptive to questions or concerns the mentee might have. This will foster a sense of trust and make the mentee more comfortable seeking guidance.

3. **Empathy**: Put yourself in the mentee's shoes and be mindful of their feelings and perspective. Remember that not everyone has the same level of experience or knowledge. Approach the review with empathy, understanding that they might be nervous or unsure about their code.

4. **Constructive Criticism**: Deliver feedback in a constructive manner, focusing on the code rather than the person. Instead of saying, "Your code is terrible," try saying, "I noticed a few areas where the code could be improved for clarity and efficiency."

TIPS FOR IMPROVING COMMUNICATION SKILLS AS A MENTOR

While some people are naturally gifted communicators, effective communication is a skill that can be learned and improved upon. Here are a few tips to enhance your communication skills as a mentor:

1. Active Listening

Listening is an essential component of effective communication. When the mentee is explaining their code or discussing their thought process, actively listen to what they are saying. Avoid interrupting or assuming you already know what they are going to say. This will help you better understand their perspective and provide more relevant feedback.

2. Ask Open-ended Questions

Instead of simply telling the mentee what they did wrong or how to fix it, ask open-ended questions to encourage critical thinking and problem-solving. For example, instead of saying, "You should have used a loop here," ask, "Have you considered using a loop in this situation? How do you think it would impact performance?"

3. Use Positive Language

Positive language can have a significant impact on the mentee's motivation and self-esteem. Instead of focusing solely on the mistakes or areas for improvement, also highlight the positive aspects of their code. For example, say, "I really like how you structured this function. It makes the code easy to read and understand."

4. Provide Context

When giving feedback or suggestions, provide context for your comments. Explain why a particular approach or solution is better and how it aligns with industry best practices. This will help the mentee understand the reasoning behind your suggestions and encourage them to learn and grow.

5. Be Mindful of Tone

Written communication can sometimes be misinterpreted, as there are no facial expressions or vocal tones to convey emotion. Be mindful of your tone and choose your words carefully to ensure your feedback is received positively. When in doubt, read your comments aloud or ask a colleague to review them for any unintentional harshness.

By improving your communication skills as a mentor, you can create a positive and productive environment during code reviews. Remember, effective communication is a two-way street, so encourage the mentee to ask questions and provide their perspective as well.

Chapter 4: Soft Skills Development

In the tech industry, it's easy to get caught up in the technical aspects of coding and forget about the importance of soft skills. But let me tell you, my friend, soft skills are like the secret sauce that takes your coding skills from good to exceptional.

So in this chapter, we're going to explore the world of soft skills development and how it can enhance your code reviews.

THE POWER OF COMMUNICATION

Picture this: You're reviewing a colleague's code and you come across a section that could be improved. Instead of bombarding them with comments and suggestions, take a step back and think about how you can communicate your feedback effectively. Remember, communication is a two-way street, and it's important to express your thoughts clearly and concisely.

One technique I like to use is the "compliment sandwich." Start off by praising something positive about the code, then provide your constructive feedback, and end with another compliment. This approach not only softens the blow of criticism but also shows that you appreciate the effort put into the code. Trust me, a little positivity can go a long way in fostering a healthy code review environment.

EMPATHY: THE KEY TO SUCCESSFUL CODE REVIEWS

Empathy is often overlooked in the tech world, but let me tell you, it's a game-changer. When you're reviewing someone's code, put yourself in their shoes and try to understand their thought process. Remember that everyone has different strengths and areas for improvement, and it's your job as a mentor to guide them in the right direction.

Instead of saying, "This code is terrible," try saying, "I see what you were trying to do here, but have you considered this alternative approach?"

By showing empathy and offering constructive suggestions, you create a safe space for growth and learning.

LEADERSHIP SKILLS: TAKING CHARGE OF CODE REVIEWS

You might be thinking, "But I'm not a manager or a team lead, why do I need leadership skills?" Well, my friend, leadership is not just about having a fancy title. It's about taking ownership and responsibility for your actions.

During code reviews, take the lead and set the tone for the review session. Encourage open and respectful discussions, and make sure everyone's voice is heard. Foster a collaborative environment where ideas are shared freely and creativity is encouraged. Trust me, when you lead by example, others will follow suit.

*PROBLEM-SOLVING ABILITIES:
TACKLING CODE ISSUES HEAD-ON*

Code reviews are not just about finding bugs or pointing out mistakes. They are also an opportunity to sharpen your problem-solving abilities. When you come across a challenging piece of code, instead of getting stuck in a loop of frustration, take a step back and think critically.

Ask yourself questions like, "What is the purpose of this code?" or "What problem is this code trying to solve?" By understanding the underlying problem, you can come up with creative solutions that not only improve the code but also enhance your problem-solving skills.

TIME MANAGEMENT: DON'T LET CODE REVIEWS DRAG ON

Ah, the dreaded time sink that is code reviews. We've all been there, spending hours going back and forth on the same piece of code. But fear not, my friend, for I have a solution for you - time management.

Set a time limit for each code review session and stick to it. This not only keeps the review focused and productive but also ensures that everyone's time is respected. If you come across a complex issue that requires more time, schedule a separate meeting to discuss it in detail. Trust me, by managing your time effectively, you'll not only become a more efficient code reviewer but also gain the respect of your colleagues.

So there you have it, my friend, the world of soft skills development in code reviews. Remember, coding is not just about writing lines of code, it's about collaborating, communicating, and growing together as a team. Embrace the power of soft skills, and watch your code reviews transform into mentoring opportunities like never before. Happy coding!

Chapter 5 - Collaborative Learning

In this chapter, we will dive into the concept of collaborative learning during code reviews. We will explore how code reviews not only benefit individual programmers but also foster a culture of collective knowledge sharing and problem-solving within a team.

THE POWER OF COLLECTIVE THOUGHT PROCESSES

Code reviews provide an opportunity for team members to come together and share their expertise. It's like a brainstorming session where different perspectives and approaches can be discussed. This collaborative environment allows for the discovery of innovative solutions and the avoidance of potential pitfalls.

Imagine a scenario where a junior programmer is stuck on a particular problem. They submit their code for review, and the team gathers to discuss it. During the review, the senior programmers share their experiences and insights, offering alternative solutions and pointing out potential issues. This collective thought process not only helps the junior programmer overcome their immediate problem but also equips them with new techniques and approaches for future challenges.

BUILDING TRUST AND TEAM COHESION

Code reviews create a platform for open and honest communication among team members. This fosters trust and strengthens the bond between team members, as they work together to improve the quality of the codebase.

When a team member submits their code for review, it's important for the reviewer to provide constructive feedback in a supportive manner. This helps create a safe environment where individuals feel comfortable sharing their work and seeking guidance. By focusing on the code rather than the person behind it, team members can avoid personal conflicts and maintain a healthy working relationship.

LEVERAGING DIVERSE SKILL SETS

One of the key benefits of collaborative learning during code reviews is the opportunity to leverage the diverse skill sets of team members. Each individual brings their own unique experiences and expertise to the table, which can greatly enrich the code review process.

For example, let's say a team is working on a complex data processing task. During the code review, a data engineering expert can provide valuable insights on optimizing the code for performance and scalability. On the other hand, a software architect can offer suggestions on improving the code's overall design and maintainability. By combining these different perspectives, the team can develop a more robust and efficient solution.

ENCOURAGING CONTINUOUS LEARNING

Code reviews should not be seen as a one-time event but rather as an ongoing process of continuous learning. By fostering a culture of collaboration and knowledge sharing, teams can create an environment where everyone is encouraged to keep learning and improving.

During code reviews, team members can share relevant resources such as articles, tutorials, or online courses that can help deepen their understanding of a particular concept or technology. Additionally, mentors can assign specific learning tasks to their mentees based on the issues identified during the review. This way, code reviews become a catalyst for personal and professional growth.

CONCLUSION

Collaborative learning is a powerful aspect of code reviews that goes beyond just catching bugs or improving code quality. It enables teams to tap into the collective knowledge and expertise of its members, fostering creativity, trust, and continuous learning. By embracing this collaborative approach, software engineering teams can elevate their skills and produce higher-quality software. So, let's embrace the power of collaboration and make our code reviews truly transformative!

Chapter 6 - Collaborative Learning

In this chapter, we will explore the concept of collaborative learning during code reviews and how these sessions can help foster problem-solving skills and build collective thought processes within a team. Code reviews should not be seen as one-sided evaluations but rather as opportunities for both the reviewer and the developer to learn from each other and improve their skills.

THE POWER OF COLLECTIVE THOUGHT

When conducting code reviews, it's essential to encourage a collaborative environment where everyone feels comfortable sharing their ideas and insights. By creating a space for open discussions, you allow for the exploration of different approaches and perspectives, leading to better problem-solving outcomes.

Imagine a scenario where a developer is struggling with a particular code implementation. During the code review, the reviewer, who has encountered a similar issue before, can offer their insights and alternative solutions. This exchange of knowledge not only helps the developer overcome their current challenge but also equips them with new skills and techniques that they can apply in future projects.

SHARING EXPERTISE

One of the most significant advantages of collaborative code reviews is the opportunity to share expertise among team members. When experienced developers participate in code reviews, they can provide valuable insights and best practices that can greatly benefit less experienced team members.

For example, let's say a junior developer has written a piece of code that works but could be optimized for performance. During the code review, a senior developer can step in and suggest alternative approaches or offer tips to improve the efficiency of the code. This not only enhances the quality of the current project but also helps the junior developer grow and learn from the experience.

BUILDING PROBLEM-SOLVING SKILLS

Code reviews provide an excellent platform for honing problem-solving skills. By encouraging discussions and brainstorming sessions during the review process, team members can collectively analyze complex problems and come up with innovative solutions.

Consider a situation where a team is facing a challenging bug that has been eluding them for days. During the code review, the team can come together to discuss the issue, share their insights, and propose potential solutions. This collaborative problem-solving approach often leads to breakthroughs and helps the team overcome obstacles more efficiently.

FOSTERING A LEARNING CULTURE

In addition to improving individual skills, collaborative code reviews help foster a learning culture within the team. When team members actively engage in discussions and share their knowledge, everyone benefits from the collective wisdom of the group.

By encouraging a learning culture, you create an environment where team members feel empowered to ask questions, seek guidance, and share their own expertise. This not only enhances individual growth but also strengthens the overall team dynamic and promotes continuous learning and improvement.

CONCLUSION

Collaborative learning during code reviews is a powerful tool for personal and professional growth. By fostering a collaborative environment, sharing expertise, and building problem-solving skills, teams can leverage the collective knowledge of their members to create superior software solutions.

In the next chapter, we will dive deeper into the concept of interpreting mistakes during code reviews and how they can be seen as opportunities for learning and growth. So buckle up and get ready for a fresh perspective on mistakes!

Chapter 7 - Constructive Feedback and Its Importance

Constructive feedback is an essential component of successful code reviews. It helps developers grow and improve their skills, while also ensuring that the team delivers high-quality code. In this chapter, we will explore the art of delivering and accepting professional feedback, and why it is crucial for the success of the code review process.

THE ART OF GIVING FEEDBACK

Giving feedback is not just about pointing out mistakes or criticizing someone's code. It is about providing constructive suggestions and offering guidance to help the developer improve. Here are some tips to master the art of giving feedback:

1. Be Specific and Actionable

When providing feedback, it's important to be specific about what needs improvement and offer actionable advice. Instead of saying, "This code is bad," provide specific examples and suggest alternative approaches. For example, you could say, "Consider using a more efficient algorithm here to improve performance."

2. Focus on the Code, Not the Person

Remember to separate the code from the developer. Instead of saying, "You made a mistake here," say, "There is an error in this section of the code." This helps create a more positive and collaborative environment, where the focus is on improving the code, not blaming individuals.

3. Use Positive Language

Constructive feedback should always be framed in a positive manner. Instead of saying, "This is wrong," try saying, "This could be improved by..." or "Have you considered..." This approach encourages the developer to view feedback as an opportunity for growth, rather than a criticism of their abilities.

4. Provide Context and Explain the Why

When giving feedback, it's important to provide context and explain the reasoning behind your suggestions. This helps the developer understand the underlying principles and make informed decisions. For example, instead of saying, "Change this variable name," explain why a more descriptive name would improve code readability and maintainability.

RECEIVING FEEDBACK WITH GRACE

Accepting feedback can sometimes be challenging, especially when it feels like a personal attack. However, learning to receive feedback with grace is essential for personal and professional growth. Here are some tips for accepting feedback:

1. Be Open-Minded

Approach feedback with an open mind and a willingness to learn. Remember that the goal of feedback is to help you improve, not to criticize your abilities. Take the feedback as an opportunity to grow and expand your knowledge and skills.

2. Don't Take it Personally

Feedback is about the code, not about you as a person. Try not to take feedback personally and avoid becoming defensive. Instead, focus on understanding the feedback and learning from it.

3. Ask for Clarification

If you don't understand a particular feedback or need more information, don't hesitate to ask for clarification. Seek to understand the reasoning behind the feedback and how it can help you improve your code.

4. Appreciate and Learn from Feedback

Show appreciation for the feedback you receive, even if it's not what you expected or wanted to hear. Every piece of feedback, whether positive or negative, is an opportunity to learn and grow as a developer. Embrace the feedback as a valuable learning experience.

Remember, the goal of constructive feedback is to foster growth and improvement, both for the individual developer and the entire team. By mastering the art of giving and receiving feedback, you can create a positive and collaborative environment that leads to better code and stronger teams.

Chapter 8 - Operating Feedback Loops: Nurturing a Culture of Continuous Improvement

In this chapter, we will delve into the importance of feedback loops in code reviews and how mentors and mentees can use them to continually assess their progress and enhance their skills. We will explore the art of delivering and accepting constructive feedback and discuss the etiquettes and best practices associated with it. So, let's dive in!

THE POWER OF FEEDBACK LOOPS

Feedback loops are essential for growth and improvement. They provide a mechanism for individuals to receive guidance, learn from their mistakes, and make necessary adjustments. In the context of code reviews, feedback loops help developers refine their coding skills, identify areas for improvement, and foster a culture of continuous learning.

As a mentor, it is crucial to establish feedback loops with your mentees. Regularly provide them with constructive feedback on their code, highlighting both the strengths and areas that need improvement. Encourage them to ask questions and seek clarification whenever needed. By actively engaging in feedback loops, you create an environment that promotes growth and development.

TEACHING "FEEDBACK ETIQUETTES"

To ensure effective feedback loops, it is essential to teach mentees the etiquettes of giving and receiving feedback. Here are some guidelines that mentors can share with their mentees:

1. Give specific and actionable feedback:

When providing feedback, be specific about the issues you have identified and suggest actionable solutions. Avoid vague or general comments that may confuse the mentee.

2. Use a constructive tone:

Feedback should always be delivered in a constructive manner. Avoid harsh or negative language that might discourage the mentee. Instead, focus on providing guidance and offering solutions.

3. Focus on the code, not the person:

During a code review, it's essential to remember that the feedback is about improving the code, not criticizing the developer. Separate the person from the code and focus on addressing the issues at hand.

4. Be receptive to feedback:

As a mentee, it is equally important to be open to receiving feedback. Listen attentively, ask questions for clarification, and be willing to learn from the feedback you receive. Remember, feedback is an opportunity for growth.

CREATING A SAFE FEEDBACK ENVIRONMENT

To foster a culture of continuous improvement, it is crucial to create a safe and non-judgmental feedback environment. Here are some strategies to achieve this:

1. Encourage a growth mindset:

Promote the idea that mistakes are opportunities for learning and growth. Emphasize that feedback is not a reflection of a person's worth but a means to enhance their skills.

2. Foster open and honest communication:

Create an atmosphere where everyone feels comfortable expressing their opinions and ideas. Encourage open discussions during code reviews, where team members can share their perspectives and provide constructive feedback.

3. Celebrate successes and learn from failures:

Acknowledge and celebrate the accomplishments of team members when they implement feedback and make improvements. Similarly, when mistakes happen, encourage open discussions to understand the root causes and identify ways to prevent similar issues in the future.

4. Lead by example:

As a mentor, demonstrate the behavior you want to see in others. Be receptive to feedback yourself, acknowledge your own mistakes, and show a willingness to learn and grow. By doing so, you set an example for others to follow.

EMBRACING CONTINUOUS LEARNING

Feedback loops should not be limited to code reviews alone. Encourage mentees to seek feedback from various sources, such as their peers, other team members, or external communities. Encourage them to participate in coding challenges, attend conferences, or join online forums to expand their knowledge and skills.

As a mentor, continually assess your mentees' progress and adjust your guidance accordingly. Provide resources, suggest learning materials, and recommend specific areas for improvement. By nurturing a culture of continuous learning, you empower your mentees to become self-sufficient and confident developers.

In conclusion, feedback loops are a vital component of code reviews and mentoring. By incorporating feedback etiquettes, creating a safe feedback environment, and promoting continuous learning, mentors can help their mentees grow and excel in their coding journey. So, embrace the power of feedback loops and watch your team thrive!

Chapter 9 - Various Techniques in Code Reviews for Mentors

In this chapter, we will explore various techniques that mentors can employ during code reviews to make them more effective and impactful. These techniques go beyond the traditional review process and provide mentors with different approaches to guide and mentor their mentees.

MONTE CARLO SIMULATION: TAKING A GAMBLE ON CODE REVIEWS

One interesting technique that mentors can use is the Monte Carlo simulation. This technique involves randomly selecting a subset of code changes to review, rather than reviewing every single line of code. By doing so, mentors can simulate the real-world scenario where not all code changes can be thoroughly reviewed due to time constraints.

Using the Monte Carlo simulation, mentors can focus on reviewing the most critical and high-impact code changes, while still providing valuable feedback to the mentee. This approach not only saves time but also teaches mentees how to prioritize their code changes and identify potential areas of improvement more effectively.

For example, let's say a mentee has made multiple code changes in a large codebase. Instead of spending hours reviewing every single line, the mentor can randomly select a subset of changes to review. This allows the mentor to focus on the most critical changes and provide feedback that is more focused and actionable.

THE HELICOPTER VIEW: RISING ABOVE THE CODE

Another technique that mentors can utilize is the helicopter view. This approach involves stepping back from the code itself and looking at the overall design and architecture of the software.

By taking a higher-level perspective, mentors can identify potential issues or improvements that may not be apparent when focusing solely on the code.

The helicopter view allows mentors to guide mentees in making more informed decisions about their code changes. They can provide insights into how the code fits into the larger system, identify potential performance bottlenecks, or suggest alternative design patterns that could improve the overall quality and maintainability of the software.

For example, imagine a mentee is working on a feature that requires significant changes to the existing codebase. Instead of solely focusing on the code changes, the mentor can take a step back and analyze how these changes may impact other parts of the system. This allows the mentor to provide guidance on how to best integrate the new feature while minimizing potential conflicts or performance issues.

COMPETITIVE PROGRAMMING APPROACH: LEVEL UP YOUR CODE REVIEWS

The competitive programming approach is another technique that mentors can leverage during code reviews. This approach involves challenging the mentee to solve coding problems or optimize existing code snippets as part of the review process. By incorporating a competitive element, mentors can encourage mentees to think critically, enhance their problem-solving skills, and learn from best practices.

This technique not only makes the code review process more engaging and interactive but also helps the mentee develop a deeper understanding of programming concepts and techniques. It encourages them to explore different solutions, analyze trade-offs, and strive for more efficient and elegant code.

For example, instead of solely reviewing the code changes, the mentor can provide the mentee with a coding problem related to the changes they have made. This allows the mentee to apply their newly acquired knowledge and showcase their problem-solving skills. The mentor can then provide feedback on the approach taken, suggest alternative solutions, and highlight areas for further improvement.

CONCLUSION

In this chapter, we explored various techniques that mentors can employ during code reviews to enhance the learning and mentoring experience for their mentees. From using Monte Carlo simulations to the helicopter view and the competitive programming approach, these techniques provide mentors with alternative ways to guide and mentor their mentees.

By incorporating these techniques into their code review process, mentors can create a more engaging and effective learning environment for their mentees. These techniques not only enhance the mentees' technical skills but also foster a sense of curiosity, critical thinking, and continuous improvement.

Remember, code reviews are not just about finding bugs or improving code quality. They are also invaluable opportunities for growth, learning, and mentorship. So, don't be afraid to think outside the box and try different techniques to make your code reviews more impactful and enjoyable for both mentors and mentees.

Chapter 10 - Situations Case Study

In this chapter, we will dive into real-life situations where a proper (or poor) code review changed the course of a progressing project. By examining these case studies, we can learn from the experiences of others and understand the impact code reviews can have on software development.

A TALE OF TWO REVIEWS

Let's start with a tale of two reviews - one that went exceptionally well and another that turned into a disaster.

The Good: Bob and Alice

Bob and Alice were working on a critical feature for their company's flagship product. Bob, being the diligent programmer that he was, decided to request a code review from Alice.

During the review, Alice not only pointed out a few minor bugs but also suggested an alternative approach to solve a performance issue. Bob, being open to feedback, implemented Alice's suggestions. The end result? The feature not only worked flawlessly but also performed significantly better than expected. Bob was ecstatic, and Alice's guidance during the code review had made a huge difference.

Lesson learned: A good code review is not just about catching bugs but also about sharing knowledge and improving the overall quality of the code. Embrace feedback and be open to alternative solutions.

The Bad: The Nitpicker

In another scenario, we have a developer who we'll call "The Nitpicker." This developer had a habit of leaving nitpicky comments on every code review they conducted. Instead of focusing on the bigger picture and providing constructive feedback, The Nitpicker would obsess over indentation, variable naming, and other minor style issues.

One unfortunate day, The Nitpicker conducted a code review for a junior developer named Alex. The review was filled with snarky comments and unnecessary criticisms. Alex, feeling demoralized and discouraged, lost confidence in their coding abilities. The project suffered as a result, with Alex becoming hesitant to contribute further.

Lesson learned: Code reviews should be a learning opportunity, not a platform for belittling others. As mentors, it's crucial to provide constructive feedback and support, rather than nitpicking trivial details. Remember, we're all on the same team, working towards a common goal.

THE BUG THAT ALMOST GOT AWAY

Imagine this: you're working on a project with tight deadlines, and the pressure is mounting. In the midst of this chaos, a critical bug manages to sneak its way into the codebase. How did this happen? Let's find out.

The Missing Null Check

Meet Sarah, a seasoned programmer with an impressive track record. One day, Sarah was assigned to fix a bug in a highly complex piece of code. Due to time constraints, she decided to skip the code review process and made the fix directly in the production code.

Unbeknownst to Sarah, her fix introduced a null reference exception that went unnoticed until it caused a major system failure. The resulting downtime cost the company a significant amount of money and damaged its reputation.

What could have been done: This situation could have been prevented if Sarah had taken the time to request a code review. A fresh pair of eyes might have caught the missing null check, preventing the bug from ever reaching production.

THE HEROIC CODE REVIEW

Now, let's shift gears and talk about a heroic code review that saved the day.

The Unintended Consequences

In a large software project, the team was working on a crucial update that involved modifying a critical algorithm. The update seemed fine on the surface, but a junior developer named Max had a gut feeling that something wasn't right. He decided to request a code review from a more experienced colleague, Emily.

During the review, Emily noticed a potential flaw in the algorithm that could have led to incorrect results under certain conditions. Thanks to Max's proactive approach and Emily's careful examination, the issue was caught before it could cause any harm. The team was saved from a potentially disastrous situation, all because of a thorough code review.

What to do in this situation: If you have a gut feeling that something might be off with your code, don't hesitate to request a code review. Trust your instincts, and remember that code reviews are there to catch potential issues before they become major problems.

CONCLUSION

These case studies highlight the immense impact code reviews can have on the success or failure of

a software project. Whether it's providing
constructive feedback, catching critical bugs, or
preventing unintended consequences, code
reviews serve as a valuable mentorship
opportunity. By embracing code reviews and
learning from the experiences of others, we can
become better programmers and build superior
quality software.

Chapter 11 - Keeping Code Reviews Fresh

Welcome to Chapter 11 of "Code reviews as a
mentoring opportunity"! In this chapter, we will
explore the importance of keeping code reviews
fresh and how to rejuvenate and re-energize your
team. Code reviews can sometimes become
monotonous and lose their effectiveness if not
approached with a fresh perspective. So let's dive
in and discover some strategies to keep the code
review process exciting and engaging!

CELEBRATE WINS

One way to keep code reviews fresh is by celebrating wins. As a mentor, it's important to acknowledge and appreciate the hard work put in by your mentee. When a code review goes well and improvements are made, take a moment to celebrate the success. This can be as simple as a virtual high-five or a shoutout in the team meeting. Celebrating wins not only boosts morale but also reinforces positive behavior and motivates the team to continue striving for excellence.

Remember, a little celebration goes a long way in creating a positive and encouraging environment for learning and growth. So don't forget to sprinkle some confetti of appreciation during your code review journey!

Another way to keep code reviews fresh is by introducing healthy challenges. Encourage your mentee to step out of their comfort zone and explore new techniques or technologies. This could involve suggesting alternative solutions or proposing creative approaches to solve a problem. By challenging your mentee, you not only push them to expand their knowledge and skills but also foster a sense of curiosity and innovation within the team.

However, it's important to strike a balance between challenging and overwhelming. Ensure that the challenges are within the mentee's capabilities and provide guidance and support throughout the process. Remember, the goal is to stretch their abilities, not break them!

CONTINUOUS IMPROVEMENT

To keep code reviews fresh, it's crucial to emphasize the importance of continuous improvement. Encourage your mentee to seek feedback not only from you but also from other team members. This can be done through peer code reviews or even informal discussions. By involving multiple perspectives, you create an environment that promotes learning and knowledge sharing.

Additionally, encourage your mentee to reflect on their own code review process and identify areas for improvement. This could involve setting personal goals, experimenting with new techniques, or even exploring different code review tools. By constantly seeking ways to improve, you ensure that the code review process remains dynamic and evolves with the changing needs of the team.

EMBRACE DIVERSITY

Lastly, to keep code reviews fresh, embrace diversity. Encourage different team members to participate in code reviews, regardless of their experience or background. By involving individuals with diverse perspectives, you introduce fresh ideas and approaches to problem-solving. This not only enriches the code review process but also fosters a culture of inclusivity and collaboration within the team.

Moreover, don't be afraid to learn from your mentee! They may bring unique insights or introduce you to new technologies or methodologies. Remember, mentoring is a two-way street, and embracing diversity ensures a constant flow of knowledge and innovation.

So there you have it - some strategies to keep code reviews fresh and exciting. By celebrating wins, introducing healthy challenges, emphasizing continuous improvement, and embracing diversity, you can maintain a vibrant and dynamic code review process. Happy reviewing!

Chapter 12 - The Power of Positive Code Reviews

Welcome to the final chapter of our book! In this chapter, we will explore the power of positive code reviews and how nurturing the right environment for coding can lead to mentally stronger software developers as well as superior quality programs. So grab your favorite beverage and let's dive in!

THE IMPACT OF POSITIVITY

Code reviews are often seen as a daunting and stressful process. Developers dread the thought of having their code scrutinized and criticized. But what if we told you that code reviews can actually be a positive experience? Yes, you heard that right!

When code reviews are conducted in a positive and supportive manner, they can have a profound impact on the team dynamics and the overall quality of the code. By fostering an environment of encouragement and constructive feedback, developers are more likely to feel motivated and inspired to write better code.

BUILDING CONFIDENCE

One of the key benefits of positive code reviews is the boost in developer confidence. When developers receive praise and recognition for their good work, it not only validates their skills but also instills a sense of pride in their abilities. This confidence then translates into better code quality as developers are more likely to take risks and explore innovative solutions.

On the other hand, negative and overly critical code reviews can have a detrimental effect on developer confidence. It can lead to self-doubt and demoralization, ultimately hampering productivity and creativity. So, as mentors, it is important for us to focus on the positive aspects of the code and provide constructive feedback that helps developers grow.

FOSTERING COLLABORATION

Positive code reviews also facilitate collaboration within the team. When developers feel comfortable sharing their code and ideas, it creates an environment of trust and camaraderie. This, in turn, leads to more open and fruitful discussions during code reviews, where team members can learn from each other and collectively improve the codebase.

Encourage developers to ask questions, seek clarification, and share their insights during code reviews. By fostering a collaborative atmosphere, you not only enhance the learning experience but also create a space where everyone feels valued and heard.

CELEBRATING WINS

Another way to infuse positivity into code reviews is by celebrating wins, no matter how small they may be. Did a developer find a clever solution to a complex problem? Did they refactor a piece of code that significantly improved performance? These achievements deserve recognition!

Taking the time to acknowledge and celebrate these wins not only boosts morale but also reinforces positive behavior. It encourages developers to continue striving for excellence and motivates others to follow suit. So, don't shy away from praising the good work and sharing success stories during code reviews.

MAINTAINING A HEALTHY BALANCE

While positivity is crucial in code reviews, it is important to strike a balance and not shy away from providing constructive feedback when necessary. It's not about sugarcoating issues or avoiding difficult conversations, but rather about delivering feedback in a way that is respectful and helpful.

Remember, constructive feedback is an opportunity for growth and improvement. So, when pointing out areas for improvement, focus on the solution rather than just highlighting the problem. Offer guidance, suggest alternative approaches, and provide resources that can help developers enhance their skills.

WRAPPING UP

And that concludes our book on "Code Reviews as a Mentoring Opportunity"! We hope that throughout this journey, you have gained valuable insights into the importance of code reviews and how they can be leveraged as a mentoring tool.

By conducting effective and positive code reviews, you have the power to transform not only the quality of the code but also the professional growth and development of your team members. So go forth, embrace the mentoring opportunity, and create a culture of learning and collaboration within your organization.

Remember, the success of code reviews lies not only in the technical aspects but also in the human element. Be kind, be supportive, and be a mentor who inspires!

Chapter 13 - The Power of Positive Code Reviews

As we reach the end of this book, it's time to explore the incredible power of positive code reviews. Throughout this journey, we have emphasized the importance of constructive feedback, mentorship, and continuous learning. However, it's equally important to create an environment that fosters positivity and encourages growth.

THE IMPACT OF POSITIVITY

When code reviews are approached with a positive mindset, it can have a profound impact on the entire team. Positive feedback not only boosts morale but also helps build confidence in developers. It creates an atmosphere where individuals feel appreciated for their efforts and are motivated to continue improving.

A Personal Experience

Let me share a personal experience to illustrate the power of positive code reviews. Back in my early days as a programmer, I was working on a complex feature for a project. I had put in countless hours, poured over documentation, and tested my code extensively. However, when it came time for the code review, I was nervous about any potential criticism.

To my surprise, my mentor approached the code review with a positive attitude. He praised the parts where I had excelled, highlighting the areas where my code was clean and efficient. He then provided constructive feedback on the areas that needed improvement, but always in a supportive and encouraging manner.

This positive approach made all the difference. Instead of feeling demoralized, I felt motivated to address the feedback and make my code even better. I realized that the goal of code reviews is not to point out flaws but to help each other grow and learn.

NURTURING A POSITIVE ENVIRONMENT

Creating a positive code review environment requires effort from everyone on the team. Here are some strategies to foster positivity:

Celebrate Wins

Take the time to celebrate successes and acknowledge the hard work put into a project. Whether it's a well-designed solution, an optimized algorithm, or an elegant piece of code, recognizing and appreciating these achievements can go a long way in boosting morale.

Encourage Collaboration

Promote a collaborative atmosphere where team members actively engage in discussions and share their knowledge. Encourage developers to ask questions, seek help, and provide assistance. By fostering collaboration, we create an environment where everyone feels valued and supported.

Provide Constructive Feedback

When providing feedback, focus on the positive aspects of the work before addressing areas for improvement. By starting the conversation on a positive note, you set the stage for a constructive discussion. Remember to be specific in your feedback and offer suggestions for improvement rather than simply pointing out flaws.

Lead by Example

As a mentor or tech leader, it's important to lead by example. Show appreciation for the efforts of your team members and provide constructive feedback in a positive and supportive manner. By setting the tone for positivity, you encourage others to adopt the same mindset.

THE RIPPLE EFFECT

The power of positive code reviews extends beyond the immediate impact on individuals. It creates a ripple effect that spreads throughout the team and the organization as a whole. When team members feel valued and supported, they are more likely to take risks, explore new ideas, and contribute to the overall success of the project.

CONCLUSION

In this book, we have explored the many facets of code reviews as a mentoring opportunity. We have discussed the basics, the role of mentors, communication skills, soft skills development, and collaborative learning. We have also delved into interpreting mistakes, delivering constructive feedback, and operating feedback loops.

Now, as we conclude this journey, let us remember the power of positive code reviews. By fostering a positive environment, celebrating wins, encouraging collaboration, and providing constructive feedback, we can create a nurturing space for software developers to thrive.

So, let's embrace the power of positivity in our code reviews and watch as our teams flourish, our software improves, and our industry grows. Together, we can create a culture of continuous learning, mentorship, and excellence. Happy coding!